I0439662

Table of Contents

I. Designated Lead Federal Agency Officials

Office of National AIDS Policy
(ONAP)

Douglas M. Brooks, MSW,
Director

Office of Management and Budget
(OMB)

Julian Harris, MD, MBA,
Associate Director for Health Programs

Department of Health and Human Services
(HHS)

Karen DeSalvo, MD, MPH,
Assistant Secretary for Health (acting)

Department of Housing and Urban Development
(HUD)

Ann Oliva,
Deputy Assistant Secretary for Special Needs
Programs

Department of Justice
(DOJ)

Vanita Gupta, JD,
Assistant Attorney General for Civil Rights (acting)

Department of Labor
(DOL)

Kathy Martinez,
Assistant Secretary for Disability Employment Policy

Department of Veterans Affairs
(VA)

Carolyn Clancy, MD,
Interim Under Secretary for Health

II. Introduction

Since President Obama released the nation's first comprehensive National HIV/AIDS Strategy in July 2010, a seismic shift in how the nation conducts HIV research, prevention, care, and treatment has occurred. Central to the Strategy is the unifying vision that "the United States will become a place where new HIV infections are rare and when they do occur, every person, regardless of age, gender, race/ethnicity, sexual orientation, gender identity or socio-economic circumstance, will have unfettered access to high quality, life-extending care, free from stigma and discrimination." Implementation of the Affordable Care Act, which has now extended health care coverage to millions of Americans, has a dynamic and evolving relationship with the Strategy that in coordination addresses the public health imperative to stop AIDS in the United States. In the nearly five years since passage of the Affordable Care Act and release of the National HIV/AIDS Strategy, the knowledge, tools and infrastructure at our disposal to prevent new infections and deliver care and services have changed dramatically (Figure 1).

The Strategy's goals are to reduce new HIV infections, increase access to care and improve outcomes for people living with HIV, and reduce HIV-related health disparities. Last year, President Obama launched the HIV Care Continuum Initiative to further the goals of the National HIV/AIDS Strategy and galvanize the national response to HIV. The initiative directs Federal agencies to step up their efforts to improve outcomes by accelerating HIV diagnosis, linkage to and engagement in medical care, initiation of antiretroviral treatment, and sustainability of viral suppression. Federal agencies have responded to this call, and this report highlights some of the progress that has been made toward achieving HIV Care Continuum goals. These successes include introducing new population-specific awareness campaigns, developing innovative care delivery models, tackling stigma, discrimination, and other barriers to care, strengthening data collection and its use to improve outcomes and monitor resource deployment, prioritizing new health research, and building capacity to improve service-delivery, particularly at the state and local levels.

Even with these advances, it remains clear that achieving our national goals requires further action: *First, it requires enhancing our effectiveness in reaching those disproportionately impacted by the epidemic and improving their health outcomes.* Data from Federal, state, and local sources suggest that less than a third of people with HIV achieve viral load suppression and accrue the full benefit of effective HIV medical care, which has the capacity not only to preserve health and extend life but also to reduce HIV transmission. In order to reduce the number of HIV infections in our country, we must focus and seize every opportunity to reduce geographic and demographic disparities in HIV care outcomes, especially among gay and bisexual men of all races and ethnicities, women and men of color, young people, transgender people, and persons living in southern states.

Second, achieving our national goals requires sustained effort in every sector. Developing and maintaining effective partnerships among Federal, state, local, and tribal governments and private-sector partners is critical to accelerating our collective progress. This report highlights several successes in these areas including improved Federal collaboration, innovative demonstration projects that have ushered in new ways of working across agencies and sectors, listening sessions held in American communities, and meetings that have brought the voices of those working in the field to the White House, leading to exciting new public-private partnerships.

Third, achieving our national goals requires detailed planning and a commitment to long term goals. Comprehensive planning is essential to design, fund and implement new programs, evaluate their outcomes, and analyze their results. It is only when these programs are fully implemented as a result of the hard work of committed frontline staff and volunteers—in the neighborhoods, clinics and settings where those in greatest need can be reached—that we will be able to ascertain the impact of programs and activities on the lives people who are at-risk for, and living with, HIV.

While this report focuses on improving outcomes along the care continuum, in order to realize the full vision of the Strategy and bend the curve of the HIV epidemic in America, we have to accelerate success through a comprehensive approach. This will include game-changing prevention tools, improved access to care through the provisions of the Affordable Care Act, enhanced capacity to monitor care continuum outcomes at the local level in order to close gaps in regionalized epidemics, directing resources to where HIV is most concentrated, and effective engagement of our non-government partners to improve outcomes for those most affected by the HIV epidemic.

Figure 1. Five Years of Progress: A New Era of HIV Prevention and Care.

Since taking office, the Obama Administration has overseen vast changes in HIV healthcare infrastructure and improving coordination throughout the Federal government. Major scientific advances during this time have provided new knowledge and tools.

October 2009	Ryan White HIV/AIDS Treatment Extension Act signed into law
January 2010	Ryan White HIV/AIDS Program begins collecting client-level data, allowing monitoring of health indicators like viral suppression by provider and client
March 2010	Affordable Care Act signed into law, improving access to health care for people living with HIV, and all Americans
July 2010	**National HIV/AIDS Strategy released**
December 2010	NIH-funded iPrEX study shows PrEP significantly reduces new HIV infections among gay and bisexual men and transgender women
March 2011	HIV care continuum concept first published by Gardner et al
August 2011	NIH-funded HIV Prevention Trials Network (HPTN) 052 shows that early treatment reduces HIV transmission risk by 96%
	CDC launches High Impact Prevention
March 2012	HHS treatment guidelines recommend HIV treatment for all persons diagnosed with HIV, regardless of CD4 count or viral load
	President Obama directs Federal agencies to address the intersection of violence against women and girls, HIV/AIDS, and gender-related health disparities
July 2012	FDA approves first medication for PrEP
August 2012	Partners PrEP and TDF2 studies find PrEP significantly reduces new HIV infections among heterosexual men and women
April 2013	U.S. Preventive Services Task Force recommends HIV screening for all adolescents and adults, making routine HIV testing a covered preventive health service under new health plans
July 2013	HIV Care Continuum Initiative is launched by Executive Order, focusing Federal action to improve outcomes from diagnosis to viral suppression
November 2013	AIDS Drug Assistance Program waiting lists reduced to zero
December 2013	President Obama announces realignment of $100 million at NIH toward HIV cure research
January 2014	New health coverage begins under the Affordable Care Act, which also prohibits denial based on pre-existing conditions and lifetime caps on coverage
May 2014	U.S. Public Health Service issues clinical practice guidelines on the use of PrEP to prevent HIV infection

III. Progress on National HIV/AIDS Strategy Goals

This report marks the second year of data available to track progress towards the 2015 National HIV/AIDS Strategy goals. _Improving Outcomes: Accelerating Progress along the HIV Care Continuum_, released in December 2013, showed progress from baseline to 2010 or 2011 for nine indicators.

New data in this report, from 2011 and 2012 for seven of the nine indicators, show that the nation has made further progress toward reaching a number of the 2015 goals of the National HIV/AIDS Strategy: increases in knowledge of HIV status among persons living with HIV, linkage to HIV medical care, and viral suppression among men who have sex with men (MSM), blacks, and Latinos. These advances are noteworthy, and still, more work remains. The data also highlight challenges and critical areas where more improvement is urgently needed.

When the National HIV/AIDS Strategy was released in July 2010, it was expected that the outlined large-scale changes would be implemented and accelerated over time. **To measure progress, a series of annual targets was established to achieve the 2015 goals. These targets were based on the expectation that change would increase as the Strategy was more fully implemented.** As shown in Figures 2 to 8, five percent of the total change was expected to be seen in the data for 2011. More change was expected in later years—20 percent in 2012, 40 percent in 2013, 70 percent in 2014, with 100 percent of the expected change being observed in 2015.

This report does not include new data on two of the indicators: 'Number of new HIV infections' and 'HIV transmission rate'. Since the first publication of HIV incidence estimates for the United States, CDC has continued to examine and refine the statistical model used to estimate incidence, meaning incidence estimates have not been available on a routine basis. CDC's National HIV Surveillance System is the primary source for monitoring HIV trends in the United States, including HIV incidence, and ensures national, state, and local programs are in the best position to mount adequate response to HIV in the United States.

While CDC's goal is to release all surveillance data expeditiously, the top priority is ensuring that the data and resulting estimates are accurate before they are released. As has been done previously with incidence estimates, CDC will release several years of data in a forthcoming report, including multiple years of data that enable a better analysis of trends, overall and for specific populations. **By June 2015, CDC expects to publish HIV incidence estimates for 2007-2012**; therefore, 2011 data for new HIV infections and transmission rate indicators are not presented in this report. In order to realize the full promise of the National HIV/AIDS Strategy, we have to use existing and forthcoming data to make the best possible decisions about the types of programs to implement, how to refine existing efforts, and the geographic areas and populations that will most benefit from increased, focused high quality HIV prevention, care and treatment services.

Figure 1 shows milestones in scientific advancement and national policy since the release of the Strategy. As the benefits of pre-exposure prophylaxis (PrEP) and "treatment as prevention" are more widely understood and implemented, rates of new infections and disparities could show major decreases. And as full implementation of the Affordable Care Act continues, millions of Americans, and thousands of people living with HIV, will acquire new and affordable health insurance coverage, sometimes for the first time. The following section provides a quantitative update on the Strategy's indicators, and describes the promising trends with each indicator in addition to the challenges we still face nationwide. Because national surveillance data do not reflect a "real-time" snapshot of the epidemic in the United States, this data cannot fully or accurately describe the status of progress in 2014; however, it does reflect some trends from baseline estimates toward the 2015 goals.

State Progress Reports Demonstrate That National Goals Are Achievable

In September 2014, CDC issued the first _State HIV Prevention Progress Report_, providing baseline data for all 50 states and the District of Columbia for six key indicators. These indicators measure outcomes along the HIV continuum of care and reflect national goals, including the National HIV/AIDS Strategy and Healthy People 2020. For each indicator, one or more states have already achieved the 2015 targets for the nation. There were wide ranging gaps in the results between states, and no state had met the national goals for all six indicators in the CDC report. Although people living in southern states were most likely to have been tested for HIV, death rates were highest among people living with HIV in southern states. Our national goals cannot be achieved without closing the gaps between states and ensuring that people living with HIV have the same opportunity to experience long, healthy lives no matter where they reside.

<u>Objective 1: Lower the annual number of new HIV infections by 25 percent</u>
The number of new HIV infections remained relatively stable, at approximately 50,000 new infections, for the last decade. As shown in Figure 2, the last year of currently available data is 2010.[1] Gay and bisexual men accounted for the largest number of new infections and were the only group in which new infections increased.[2]

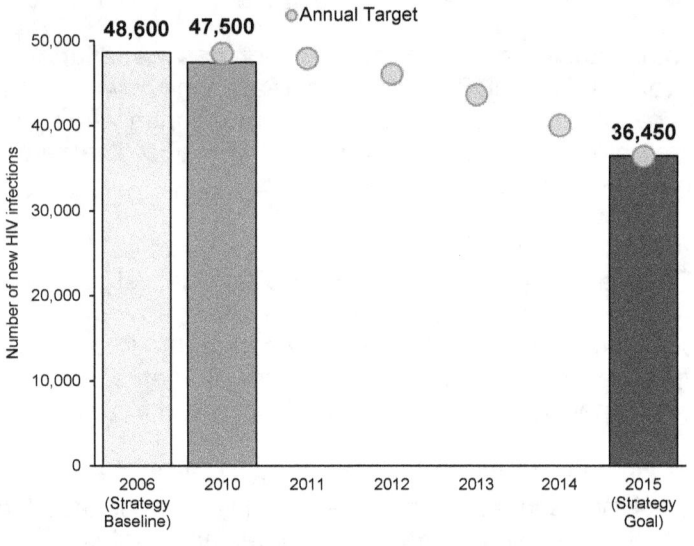

Figure 2. Annual number of new HIV infections.

Ongoing Federal action to reduce new infections:

- **Combination Prevention Strategies:** A combination of effective HIV prevention strategies, directed to the appropriate populations and geographic areas, is essential. This approach involves intensive efforts to increase HIV diagnosis, linkage and retention in care to increase viral suppression, increased awareness of and access to all proven prevention tools (including condoms and PrEP), support services for people living with and at-risk for HIV, as well as basic education for the general public.
- **Pre-exposure prophylaxis:** PrEP, the use of antiretrovirals to prevent HIV infection, is a promising strategy to complement existing prevention methods. The U.S. Public Health Service released Clinical Practice Guidelines for PrEP; subsequently, CDC and HRSA funded a PrEPLine to answer clinicians' questions about the use of PrEP for their patients.

To reach the 2015 goal, prevention efforts, including PrEP and other evidence-based strategies, must continue to be prioritized alongside the HIV continuum of care.

<u>Objective 2: Increase the percentage of people living with HIV who know their serostatus to 90 percent</u>
The number of people living with undiagnosed HIV infection has continued to decrease. In 2011, 1.2 million people were living with HIV in the United States. The percentage of persons living with HIV who know their serostatus increased from 80.9 percent in 2006 to 86.0 percent in 2011.

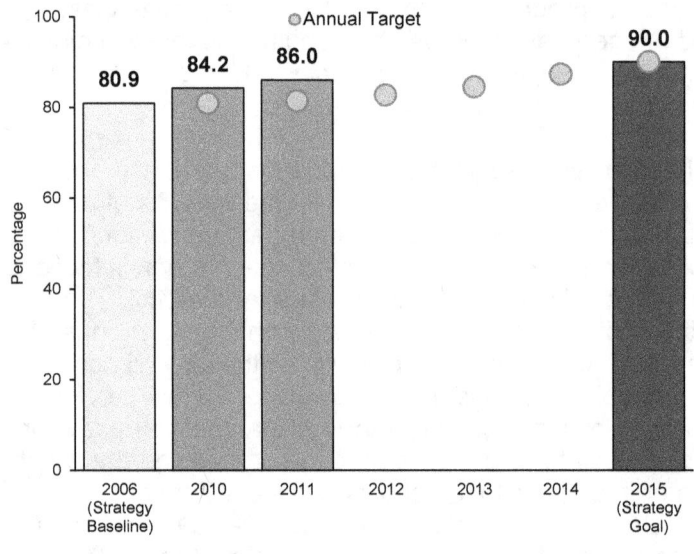

Figure 3. Annual percentage of serostatus knowledge.

Promising trends
From 2006 to 2011, the number of people living with HIV whose infection had not been diagnosed decreased by 16 percent.
More than 90 percent of people who inject drugs, and adults age 45 and older, who are living with HIV have had their infection diagnosed.
Challenges
Approximately 168,000 people are living with undiagnosed HIV infection in the United States.
Young persons living with HIV (aged 13 to 24 years) are less likely than older adults to know their status. Only 49 percent of young people living with HIV have been diagnosed.
Across risk groups, heterosexual men, and gay and bisexual men living with HIV are least likely to know their serostatus.

---

1. CDC. Estimated HIV incidence in the United States, 2007–2010. HIV Surveillance Supplemental Report. 2012; 17(4). Available at http://www.cdc.gov/hiv/surveillance/resources/reports/2010supp_vol17no4/.
2. Ibid.

Ongoing Federal actions to increase knowledge of serostatus:

- **HIV testing under the Affordable Care Act:** Under the Affordable Care Act, new health plans are required to cover HIV testing as recommended by the USPSTF without cost sharing.
- **Implementing USTSPF recommendations:** Steady progress continues to be made each year, but to reach the 2015 target, we need to ensure greater uptake of the U.S. Preventive Services Task Force (USPSTF) recommendations for HIV testing in health care settings and make certain that community-based testing reaches those at greatest risk.
- **Conducting HIV testing:** In 2012, Federal agencies with substantial supporting roles in the delivery of HIV prevention and care services[3] conducted more than nine million HIV tests and newly diagnosed more than 15,000 HIV infections.
- **Outreach to expand testing efforts:** Federal agencies have promoted HIV testing as part of *Act Against AIDS* and other public education campaigns; realigned community-based organization funding to increase HIV testing; provided information, tools and training to doctors, nurses and other health care providers; supported research to improve HIV testing; issued guidance on the use of more sensitive HIV tests to diagnose HIV infection earlier; and expanded HIV testing in community health centers, substance abuse treatment facilities, behavioral health programs and other settings.

Objective 3: Reduce the HIV transmission rate by 30 percent

The HIV transmission rate measures the number of new HIV infections in a given year per 100 people living with HIV. It is an important measure of progress because it takes into account increases in the number of people living with HIV. In 2010, the last year of available data, the transmission rate was 4.2.

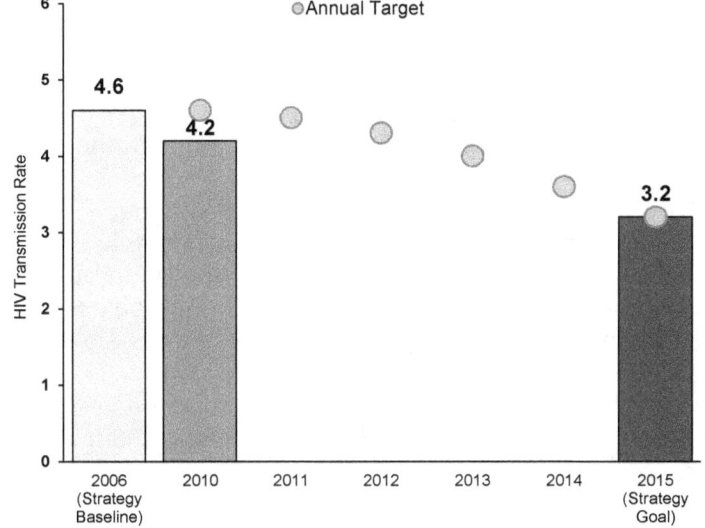

Figure 4. Annual HIV transmission rate.

Ongoing Federal action to reduce transmission rate:

- **HIV Treatment Works Campaign:** To achieve the 2015 target, the prevention benefits of people with HIV consistently taking their treatment will need to be promoted.[4] In 2014, CDC in collaboration with HRSA, launched the *HIV Treatment Works* campaign to support informed treatment and care decision-making for persons living with HIV and promote improvement in HIV care continuum outcomes.
- **Interagency Collaboration to focus on Increasing Access to Care:** HRSA collaborated with DOJ and other Federal agencies to develop the newsletter titled, *Quality In Action: Increasing Access to HIV Testing, Care, Treatment*, which described strategies that health centers and free clinics can use to increase the number of people aware of their HIV status and ensure that people living with HIV get the full benefits of care and treatment.

Objective 4: Increase the percentage of persons diagnosed with HIV who are linked to HIV medical care within three months of diagnosis to 85 percent

All people diagnosed with HIV should be linked to high-quality medical care and support services promptly following diagnosis. This ensures that their health is properly evaluated and they can begin the care and treatment that is necessary to live a longer, healthier life with HIV, and also prevent the transmission of HIV to others. Comprehensive medical care should be a portal for connecting people with other services (such as mental health support, substance abuse treatment, and housing) and helping individuals overcome personal barriers to successful HIV treatment.[5]

---

3. Excludes information about HIV testing supported by the Department of Defense and the Department of Justice.
4. Cohen, M.S., et al. Prevention of HIV-1 Infection with Early Antiretroviral Therapy. New England Journal of Medicine. 2011; 365: 493–505.
5. White House Office of National AIDS Policy. National HIV/AIDS Strategy for the United States, July 2010.

Figure 5. Percentage of HIV-diagnosed persons linked to care.

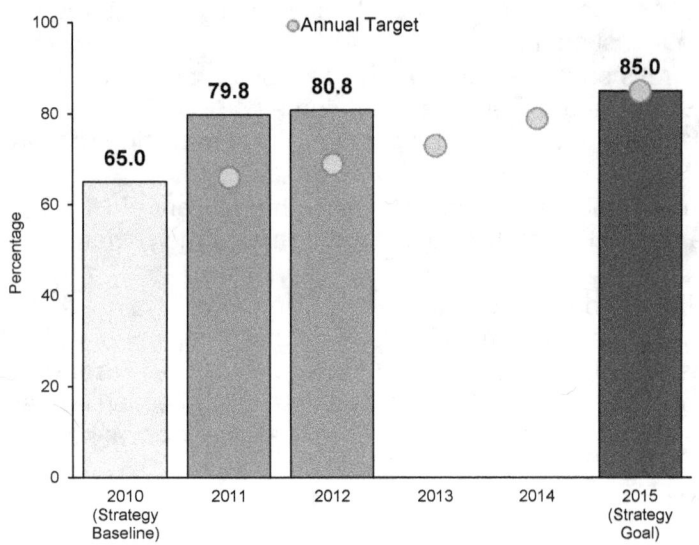

<table>
<tr><td colspan="3" align="center">**Promising trends**</td></tr>
<tr><td colspan="3">The 2015 target was met in 2012 for Native Hawaiian and other Pacific Islanders, whites, persons of multiple races, and those 55 years of age or older.</td></tr>
<tr><td colspan="3">Seven states (Iowa, New Hampshire, North Dakota, South Carolina, Utah, West Virginia, and Wyoming) and the District of Columbia met or exceeded the 2015 target in 2012.</td></tr>
<tr><td colspan="3" align="center">**Challenges**</td></tr>
<tr><td colspan="3">Fewer than 80 percent of newly diagnosed blacks, American Indians/Alaskan Natives, people who inject drugs, heterosexual men, and those aged 13 to 24 years were linked to care within 3 months.</td></tr>
<tr><td colspan="3">Results vary widely between states, and too few states report complete laboratory data that are needed to monitor progress along the HIV care continuum.[6]</td></tr>
</table>

Ongoing Federal actions to increase linkage to care:

- **Increased access to testing and prevention**: In 2014, Federal agencies and their partners have worked to implement new programs and modify existing programs to improve linkage to HIV medical care. CDC announced the availability of $210 million to support up to 100 community-based organizations for a 5-year project that will increase access to HIV testing and prevention in communities that are most heavily affected by HIV and improve outcomes along the HIV care continuum.

- **High-Impact Prevention**: CDC has also re-directed $40 million in HIV prevention funds to support Community High-Impact Prevention, a new strategy to assist community-based organizations and capacity building assistance providers in targeting resources toward prevention strategies with the highest impact that further goals of the HIV Care Continuum Initiative.

- **Improving access to community health centers**: HHS invested $11 million to enhance HRSA-funded community health centers to support the integration of HIV into primary care within in communities highly impacted by HIV, especially among racial and ethnic minorities. This initiative, funded through the Affordable Care Act and the Secretary's Minority AIDS Initiative Fund (SMAIF), aims to build sustainable partnerships between public health and primary care health centers and support expanded HIV Service delivery to help achieve the goals of the Strategy.

- **Research on best practices**: NIH and other agencies are funding research that will yield information to help HIV testing providers successfully link persons newly diagnosed with HIV to medical care in a timely manner.

Objective 5: Increase the percentage of Ryan White program clients in continuous care to 80 percent[7]
Federal guidelines for the use of Antiretroviral Agents in HIV-1 infected Adults and Adolescents now recommend that all adults and adolescents living with HIV in the United States be offered antiretroviral treatment.[8] This fosters an even more urgent need to engage people diagnosed with HIV who have never been in care or who have subsequently fallen out of care. There is also a need for ongoing support to maintain high levels of adherence to antiretroviral treatment.[9]

---

6. HRSA HIV/AIDS Bureau. The Ryan White HIV/AIDS Program Progress Report 2012: Ahead of the Curve. November 2012.
7. In the Strategy, continuous care is defined as at least two visits for routine HIV medical care in 12 months at least three months apart.
8. NIH. Guidelines for the Use of Antiretroviral Agents in HIV-1-Infected Adults and Adolescents. Available at http://www.aidsinfo.nih.gov/guidelines.
9. White House Office of National AIDS Policy. National HIV/AIDS Strategy for the United States, July 2010

Figure 6. Percentage of Ryan White clients in continuous care.

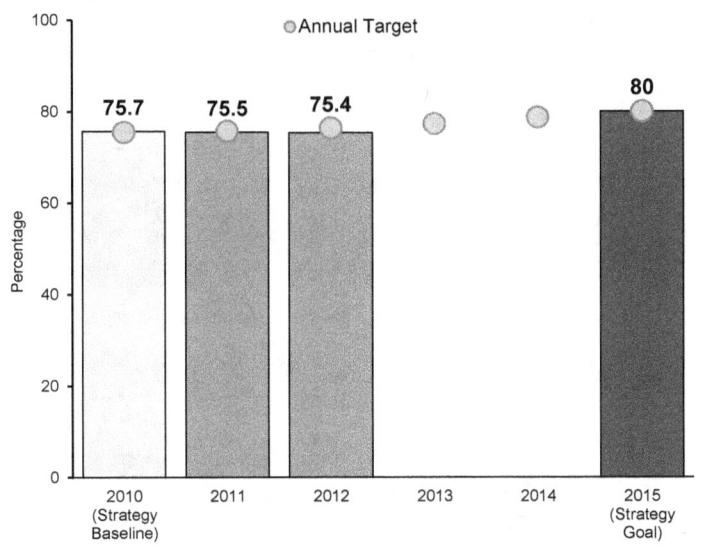

	Promising trends	
Overall, three out of four Ryan White clients were in continuous HIV medical care. Among Ryan White clients, there were few differences in continuous care by race/ethnicity (74.7 percent white; 74.2 percent black; 79.3 percent Latino). Data from 2012 suggest that women have better retention in care outcomes (77.1 percent) compared to men (74.9 percent).		
There were few differences by risk group (75.4 percent MSM, 76.5 percent heterosexual, 76.2 percent IDU).		

Challenges
Transgender Ryan White clients (72.6 percent) had lower rates of continuous care compared to cisgender men (74.9 percent) or women (77.1 percent).
Young adults aged 19 to 24 years had that lowest percentage of continuous care (64.1 percent), followed by those aged 25 to 34 years (68.9 percent).[10]

Ongoing Federal actions to increase Ryan White clients in continuous care:

- **Improving Data Collection:** The Ryan White HIV/AIDS Program has developed data systems to more accurately measure those in continuous care. HRSA will track data on a client level, providing insights into how care is accessed and the impact on viral load suppression.
- **Increasing Access through the Affordable Care Act:** With implementation of the Affordable Care Act, more people living with HIV have access to affordable healthcare coverage.
- **Improving Coordination:** Ryan White program grantees, Medicaid programs, CDC-funded surveillance programs, medical providers, and community-based organizations are strengthening coordination to support and monitor engagement in care.

Objective 6: Increase the percentage of Ryan White program clients with permanent housing to 86 percent

Access to stable housing is an important precursor to engaging in regular care. Homeless or marginally housed people living with HIV are more likely to delay or have poorer access to care and are less likely to receive and adhere to optimal antiretroviral therapy.[11]

Promising trends
Most Ryan White clients were stably housed from 2010-2012. Since baseline, the percentage of Ryan White clients with permanent housing increased from 82 to 84.5 percent. Those over 65 years of age were the most stably housed compared to all other age groups at 84.7 percent.

Challenges
In 2012, Hispanic and transgender clients were least likely to report stable housing (77.1 percent and 68.6 percent, respectively).
From 2010 to 2012 there was only a modest increase in the percent of Ryan White clients that were stably housed.

Figure 7. Percentage of Ryan White clients with permanent housing.

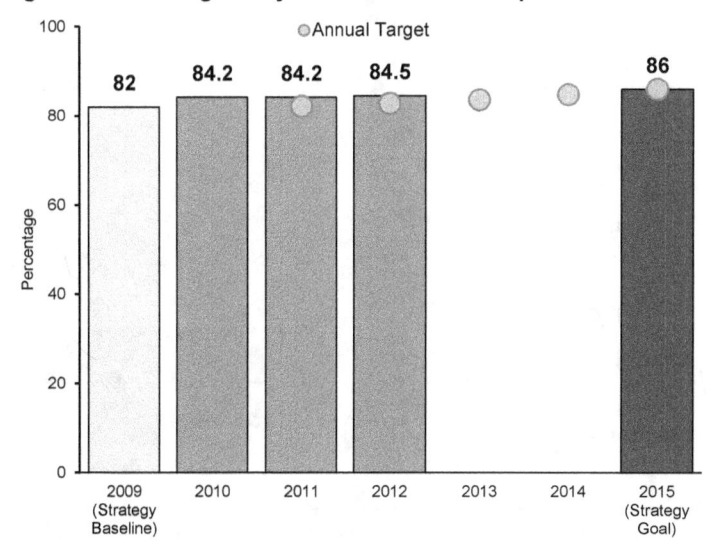

---

10. HRSA HIV/AIDS Bureau. The Ryan White HIV/AIDS Program Progress Report 2012: Ahead of the Curve. November 2012.
11. Aidala AA, et al. Housing need, housing assistance, and connection to medical care. AIDS Behav 2007; 11 (supp2); S101-S115.

Ongoing Federal actions to increase Ryan White clients with permanent housing:

- **HOPWA focus on Integrated Services:** A substantial majority of Ryan White program patients are stably housed. The Department of Housing and Urban Development's (HUD) Housing Opportunities for Persons with AIDS (HOPWA) program's new emphasis on integrating housing and care services will strive to improve outcomes along the HIV Care Continuum.
- **Maximizing Employment Opportunities:** The Department of Labor's (DOL) support of policies and practices to maximize employment opportunities for people living with HIV marks important steps towards increasing housing stability for people living with HIV. In 2014, the DOL and HUD launched *Getting to Work: A Training Curriculum for HIV/AIDS Service Providers and Housing Providers*.

<u>Objectives 7, 8, and 9: Increase the percentages of HIV-diagnosed MSM, blacks and Latinos with a suppressed viral load by at least 20 percent</u>

Increasing viral suppression among the population groups that are hardest hit by HIV is essential for improving the health and well-being of people living with HIV and preventing new HIV infections. Gay, bisexual, and other men who have sex with men, blacks, and Latinos, and subpopulations within those groups, share disproportionate burdens of new HIV infections, compared to their percentage of the overall population.[12] By increasing viral suppression rates and decreasing community viral load in these specific populations, not only does individual health improve, but the potential for substantial reductions in new HIV infections also improves.[13]

Figure 8. Percentage of MSM, blacks, and Latinos (respectively) with suppressed viral load.

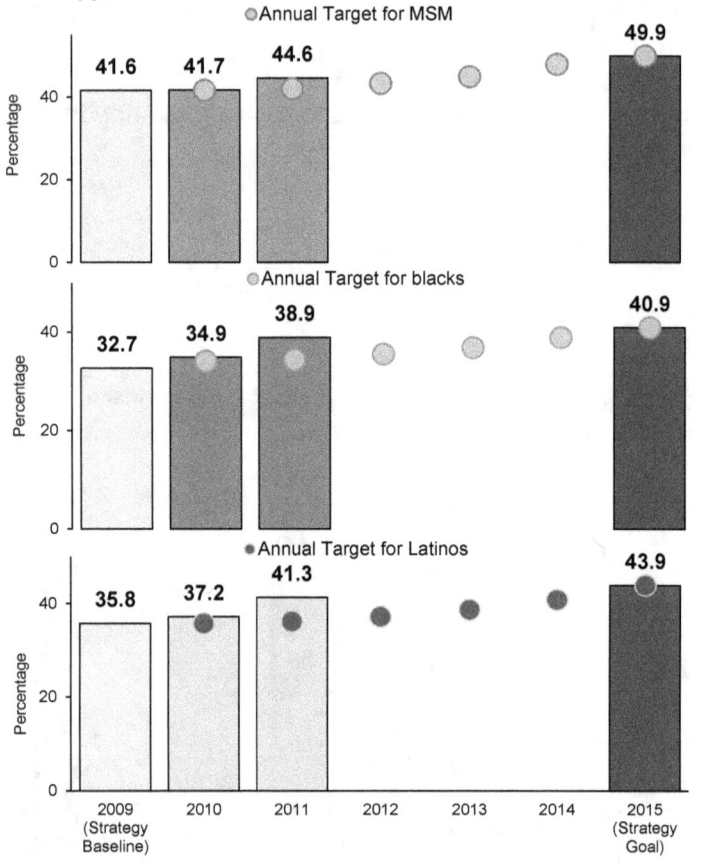

Promising results
Improvements in viral suppression were seen for all three groups.
Compared to the 2009 baseline, viral suppression increased 19 percent among blacks, 15 percent among Latinos, and 7 percent among MSM.

Challenges
Increasing viral suppression will require improvements along the entire HIV care continuum, especially HIV diagnosis and on-going engagement in HIV medical care.
Fewer than half of MSM, blacks and Latinos who have been diagnosed with HIV have achieved viral suppression.[14]

12. Monitoring selected national HIV prevention and care objectives by using HIV surveillance data—United States and 6 dependent areas—2012. HIV Surveillance Supplemental Report 2014; 19(No.3). http://www.cdc.gov/hiv/library/reports/surveillance/index.html. Published November 2014.

13. Das M, et al. "Decreases in community viral load are accompanied by reductions in new HIV infections in San Francisco." PloS One 5.6. 2010; e11068.

14. Monitoring selected national HIV prevention and care objectives by using HIV surveillance data—United States and 6 dependent areas—2012. HIV Surveillance Supplemental Report 2014; 19(No.3). http://www.cdc.gov/hiv/library/reports/surveillance/index.html. Published November 2014.

Helping People with HIV Reach Quality Health Outcomes through the Ryan White Program

In 2012, the Ryan White HIV/AIDS Program served approximately 536,000 low-income people with HIV in the United States. HRSA reports that the Ryan White HIV/AIDS Programs served 52 percent of the estimated persons that are living with diagnosed HIV infection. The Ryan White HIV/AIDS Program can measure the impact of its actions through client level data. Most recent data for services provided from 2010 to 2012 demonstrate that those who are retained in Ryan White medical care increased viral suppression rates from 69.5 percent in 2010 to 75.1 percent in 2012, due in part to increased investments in the AIDS Drug Assistance Program and increased technical assistance activities. In addition, ADAP waiting lists decreased from a peak of 9,310 in September 2011 to zero in September 2014. In FY 2012, more than 244,436 persons received HIV-related medications through the ADAP, the nation's treatment safety net for persons living with HIV.

Ongoing Federal actions to increase viral suppression:

- **Reducing waitlists for ADAP:** HRSA has made major progress in the care and outcomes of the people living with HIV that it serves. Viral suppression has increased among Ryan White clients and waitlists for AIDS Drug Assistance Programs (ADAPs) have been eliminated around the country.

- **Integration of Behavioral Health with HIV services:** In 2014, SAMHSA funded an important new project, the *Minority AIDS Initiative Care Pilot: Integration of HIV Medical Care Into Behavioral Health Programs*, which over four years, will integrate a comprehensive set of behavioral health and medical care services in substance abuse and community mental health programs that serve racial and ethnic minority populations at high risk for behavioral health disorders and HIV.

- **Increased testing and engagement in care among vulnerable populations:** Agencies across HHS, VA and HUD are working to encourage HIV testing among gay and bisexual men, blacks and Latinos, and to counter myths about HIV medical care and treatment, and to educate people living with HIV about their rights. For example, the HHS Office of Civil Rights and its partners are educating people living with HIV through the *Information is Powerful Medicine* campaign. SMAIF has provided funding to HRSA to support the National Alliance of State and Territorial AIDS Directors to enhance the capacity of Ryan White program grantees to increase the engagement and retention of young gay men of color in HIV medical care. VA expanded HIV testing programs among homeless Veterans around the country.

We have already seen important signs of progress as a result of implementing the National HIV/AIDS Strategy at the Federal and local levels. Scientific and programmatic advances in HIV prevention and care mean that we have the tools to achieve the goals of the Strategy. But much important work remains to be done to achieve our nation's vision of an AIDS-free generation. If we work together to strengthen our partnerships, galvanize state and local responses, and steer resources to those most affected by HIV, we can maximize our collective impact and fully realize the goals of the National HIV/AIDS Strategy.

IV. Progress on Implementing HIV Care Continuum Initiative Recommendations

Much has been accomplished at the Federal, state, and local levels toward improving outcomes across the HIV Care Continuum. At the Federal level, new data and the implementation of new programs reflect the focus on improving care along the spectrum from diagnosis to viral suppression.

New data in Figure 9 released by CDC show improvement on some care continuum outcomes.[15] In 2011, of the estimated 1.2 million persons living with HIV infection in the United States, an estimated 86 percent were aware of their infection. Among the more than 15,000 persons newly diagnosed with HIV infection in 2011, 80 percent were linked to HIV medical care within 3 months after diagnosis. Among the 1.2 million persons living with HIV infection in 2011, 40 percent were engaged in HIV medical care, 37 percent were prescribed antiretroviral therapy (ART), and 30 percent achieved viral suppression. The percentage of people living with HIV who achieved viral suppression in 2011 (30 percent) was roughly stable compared to the updated estimates for 2009 (26 percent).[16]

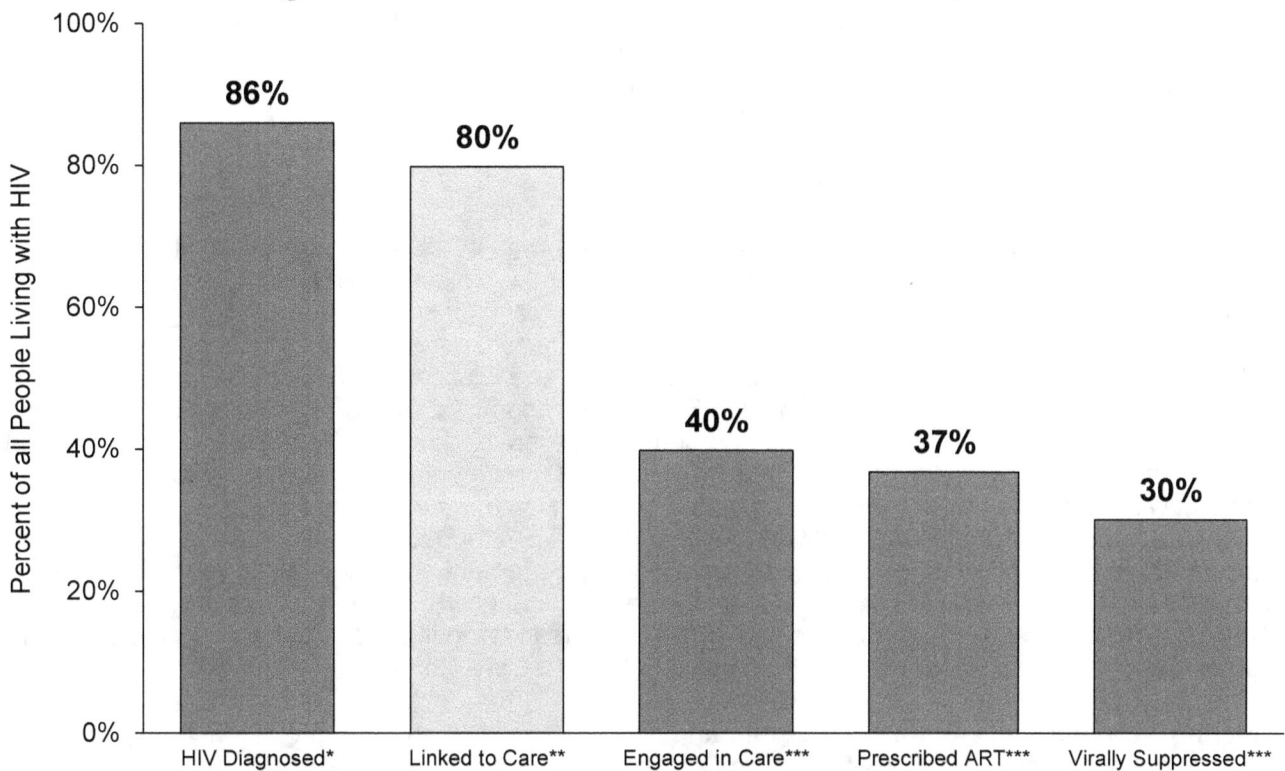

Figure 9. The HIV Care Continuum in the United States, 2011.

* Diagnosed is a calculated estimate based on data reported to the National HIV Surveillance System, the denominator is the estimated number of persons living with HIV (1.2 million).
** Linkage to care was calculated based on percentage of persons newly diagnosed in 2011 (n=15,499) that were linked to medical care (12,333) within 3 months after diagnosis.
*** Engaged in care, prescribed ART and virally suppressed data come from the Medical Monitoring Project (MMP) and are based on people who had at least one visit during 2011. The dominator is the estimated number of persons living with HIV (1.2 million).

---

15. Since it was first published in 2011, the HIV care continuum has been used widely, but displayed with various data sources and different measures for each of the outcomes along the continuum. Some of the changes in the continuum over time were based on increased availability of data; other differences in how the continuum is displayed reflect how each of the care continuum outcomes are measured, or what number is used in the denominator. In this report, for example, Figure 9 shows the data for linkage to care in a different colored bar from the other outcomes due to it being measured only for persons diagnosed during 2011 in selected states while the other outcomes are measured for the 1.2 million people living with HIV infection in the US.

16. CDC. Monitoring Selected National HIV Prevention and Care Objectives by Using HIV Surveillance Data, United States and 6 Dependent Areas, 2012. HIV Surveillance Supplemental Report 2014; 19 (No.3).

These new care continuum data show that 6 in 7 people with HIV know their status and that 8 in 10 of those who were newly diagnosed with HIV in 2011 were linked to HIV medical care within 90 days. Notably, they demonstrate an important detail that once people are engaged in medical care, the majority achieve the ultimate outcome: viral suppression. However, the data also point to the urgent need to reach more people with HIV testing, and ensure those who test positive receive prompt, ongoing care and treatment. Our efforts to accelerate outcomes along each step of the care continuum, at the Federal level and otherwise, are imperative to improve each of its bars.

In response to the HIV Care Continuum Working Group recommendations released in December 2013, Federal agencies have made progress in funding new initiatives, research, implementing programs, and providing assistance to state and local governments and communities to improve each of these bars along the care continuum. Below are specific highlights of actions Federal agencies took this year to address the HIV care continuum by expanding and refocusing programs, reducing stigma and discrimination, building capacity at the state and local levels, and integrating services that could break down barriers to accessing care and ultimately improve outcomes along the continuum.

- **Providing analysis and guidance on HIV-specific state criminalization laws:** In March 2014, DOJ, in collaboration with CDC, published an analysis that examined HIV-specific state laws, and the risk of HIV transmission by type of activities engaged in.[17] There are 33 states that have one or more HIV specific laws that criminalize behaviors that the CDC regards as posing either no or negligible risk for HIV transmission. These laws further stigmatize HIV and those living with HIV. DOJ published a follow-up document in July 2014 titled *Best Practices Guide to Reform HIV-Specific Criminal Laws to Align with Scientifically-Supported Factors* to provide guidance and technical assistance to states that wish to ensure that their existing policies do not place unique or additional burdens on individuals living with HIV/AIDS and that policies reflect the science of HIV transmission routes and associated benefits of treatment.

- **Funding collaborative efforts to improve outcomes along the HIV care continuum at the state and local levels:** In 2014, HHS SMAIF funds were used to establish a new project co-led by CDC and HRSA's Bureau of Primary Health Care called the Partnerships for Care (P4C): Health Departments and Health Centers Collaborating to Improve HIV Outcomes. This project supports collaborations between state health departments and HRSA-funded health centers to expand and improve HIV medical care. Additionally, CDC funded the Cooperative Re-Engagement Controlled Trial (CoRECT), a randomized clinical trial of the data to care strategy of using surveillance and clinic data to identify persons out of care and re-engage them in care. CDC has announced the availability of $210 million to support up to 100 community-based organizations for a 5-year project that will increase access to HIV testing and prevention in communities that are most heavily affected by HIV and improve outcomes along the HIV care continuum. HRSA funded a new initiative to enhance the capacity of Ryan White program grantees to increase the engagement and retention of young gay men of color in care. CDC has also re-directed $40 million in HIV prevention funds to support Community High-Impact Prevention, a new strategy to assist CBOs and CBA providers in targeting resources toward the prevention strategies with the highest impact that furthers goals of the HIV Care Continuum Initiative.

- **Integrating behavioral health into HIV Services:** In 2014, SAMHSA created the Minority AIDS Initiative Continuum of Care Pilot-Integration of HIV Medical Care into Behavioral Health Programs. The purpose of this four year program is to integrate care (behavioral health treatment, prevention, and HIV medical care services) for racial/ethnic minority populations at high risk for behavioral health disorders and at high risk for or living with HIV. This program is primarily intended for substance abuse treatment programs and community mental health programs that can co-locate and/or fully integrate HIV prevention and medical care services. This program will encourage behavioral health screening, primary substance abuse and HIV prevention, substance abuse, mental health, and co-occurring treatment, creation of infrastructure to provide integrated care, and screen for HIV and hepatitis, and provide hepatitis vaccination. It is expected that effective person-centered treatment will reduce the risk of HIV transmission, improve outcomes for those living with HIV, and ultimately reduce new infections.

---

17. Lehman JS, Carr MH, Nichol AJ, Ruisanchez A, Knight DW, Langford AE, Mermin JH. Prevalence and public health implications of state laws that criminalize potential HIV exposure in the United States. AIDS and Behavior. 2014; 18(6), 997-1006.

Federal agencies have implemented new programs and taken a wide range of actions in response to the HIV Care Continuum. The following table provides a summary of progress on each action step that the Interagency HIV Care Continuum Federal Working Group released in the 2013 report. Presented here is a summary of some of the activities that Federal agencies have completed or that are in process to improve care continuum outcomes.

Recommendation 1: Support, implement and assess innovative models to more effectively deliver care along the care continuum

Action	Federal Agency Activities
1.1 Support models of care that provide incentives for improvements along the care continuum	• HRSA linked Ryan White program defined services to each measure in the HIV care continuum to provide grantees with guidance to ensure their programs support the care continuum. HRSA also began reviewing PEPFAR best-practice models of care where incentives have been used to develop such care and make improvements along the care continuum. • HRSA initiated development of performance-based metrics and incentives to determine future awards and grantees, and funded a project to support a learning collaborative that will cut across all 52 Part A jurisdictions in measuring and making improvements along the HIV care continuum. • Under the Affordable Care Act, states are creating health homes intended to better coordinate care for people with Medicaid. CMS is now supporting 20 health homes in 16 states, and in particular, four states have health homes to address the needs of more than 50,000 beneficiaries living with HIV.
1.2 Promote the use of real-time routine electronic HIV clinical reminders at all VA facilities to increase HIV testing among veterans	• HIV Clinical Reminder has been offered for use at all VA Medical Centers. Over 80 percent of facilities have already volunteered to implement the routine HIV testing clinical reminder. Those facilities that have used the clinical reminder have seen exponential increases in HIV testing rates compared to facilities that do not use the clinical reminder. VA has shared the HIV testing clinical reminder template with IHS for use throughout another Federal health care system.
1.3 Increase the capacity of Ryan White program grantees to increase the engagement and retention of young gay men of color in care	• HRSA funded a new initiative to enhance the capacity of Ryan White program grantees to increase the engagement and retention of young gay men of color in care, and will inventory existing evidence-based interventions for care and prevention using national epidemiological data as a guide to develop models of care, toolkits, and webinars which can be replicated and implemented across the care continuum for black MSM. Additionally, the project will identify and disseminate broadly best practices, evidence-based interventions, and effective models of care to HIV/AIDS providers, health centers and health departments, Federal and non-Federal HIV/AIDS stakeholders to increase their capacity to serve, enhance quality of care, and improve health outcomes for the targeted population.
1.4 Support and rigorously evaluate the development and implementation of new integrated behavioral health models to address the intersection of substance use, mental health, and HIV.	• SAMHSA, with input from HRSA, CDC and HUD, created the four-year Minority AIDS Initiative Continuum of Care Pilot-Integration of HIV Medical Care into Behavioral Health Programs to integrate care (behavioral health treatment and HIV medical care services) for racial and ethnic minority populations at high risk for behavioral health disorders and at-high-risk for or living with HIV infection. This program is intended for substance abuse treatment programs and community mental health programs that can co-locate and/or fully integrate HIV prevention and medical care services.

Recommendation 2: Tackle misconceptions, stigma and discrimination to break down barriers to care

Action	Federal Agency Activities
2.1 Develop a multimedia campaign for persons living with HIV to: 1) address myths surrounding HIV treatment; 2) reach persons who have been diagnosed, but have not been linked to care; 3) re-engage those who have dropped out of care.	• CDC, in collaboration with HRSA, developed and launched the "HIV Treatment Works" campaign to improve HIV care continuum outcomes among people living with HIV, with goals of 1) increasing engagement and retention in care and adherence to antiretroviral treatment for people living with HIV; 2) increasing information-seeking about HIV care and treatment among people with HIV; and 3) supporting informed treatment and care decision-making for people with HIV. • IHS partnered with CDC to enhance American Indian and Alaska Native inclusion in two national HIV media campaigns, "Start Talking. Stop HIV." and "Let's Stop HIV Together." The two agencies worked together to identify American Indian and Alaska Native community concerns, develop a list of potential models/ spokespeople, and conduct outreach to community stakeholders.
2.2 Issue best practice recommendations to help ensure that Federal and state criminal laws reflect current scientific knowledge regarding HIV and avoid imposition of unique or unwarranted barriers and penalties, including criminal penalties, based on HIV status.	• DOJ released *Best Practices Guide to Reform HIV-Specific Criminal Laws to Align with Scientifically-Supported Factors*, a guide for states to consider when evaluating their HIV-specific criminal statutes. Since the President's National HIV/AIDS Strategy was announced in July 2010, the Department has settled 13 cases of HIV discrimination. Two of those settlements were just reached this year, and at least 16 investigations of HIV discrimination are on-going.
2.3 Review social marketing and education campaigns related to the care continuum and incorporate nondiscrimination and Health Information Privacy messages.	• DOL and HUD, in collaboration with DOJ, incorporated nondiscrimination and Health Information Privacy information, resources, and messaging in the *Getting to Work Curriculum*, which also addresses the care continuum. • HHS Office of Civil Rights (OCR) developed and implemented the "Information is Powerful Medicine" campaign, which empowers those living with HIV to be pro-active in their medical care. These resources will be shared with other agencies to help disseminate health information privacy messages. HHS OCR also provides technical assistance regarding nondiscrimination and health information privacy messaging in public outreach campaigns under development. • A "Know Your Rights" webpage was added to the VA's National HIV Program website. DOJ reviewed all relevant VA HIV social marketing, educational campaign materials, and nondiscrimination messages. • HRSA worked with DOJ and other federal agencies to develop a newsletter, *Quality In Action: Increasing Access to HIV Testing, Care, Treatment*, which reviewed strategies that health centers and free clinics can use to increase the number of people aware of their HIV status and ensure that people living with HIV get the full benefits of care and treatment. Strategies included identifying ways to ensure health care environments are welcoming, supportive, and free of stigma and discrimination. • HUD launched a Twitter page (@HUD_HOPWA) to be used as a platform to disseminate anti-discrimination messaging related to housing. A listserv message focusing on HIV Discrimination and Housing will be disseminated to all subscribers of the HOPWA mailing list, AIDS.gov blog, and HOPWA Twitter followers.

Action	Federal Agency Activities
2.4 Conduct compliance reviews of health care providers to ensure their compliance with relevant provisions of HIPAA, and provide technical assistance to health care providers with regard to requirements to care for persons living with HIV, in compliance with Federal nondiscrimination laws.	• HHS OCR initiated compliance reviews to identify policies and practices regarding non-discrimination and health privacy messages. Hospitals under review are located in areas that serve predominately disadvantaged communities in the 12 cities most impacted by HIV/AIDS, and are being evaluated for 1) equal access to services and programs for individuals with HIV/AIDS; 2) meaningful access to services for limited English proficient (LEP) individuals, focusing on LEP individuals seeking HIV testing and counseling; 3) the privacy of individuals' protected health information; and 4) individuals' rights to their protected health information. OCR will provide technical assistance and identify effective practices on nondiscrimination, privacy and security of protected health information, and efforts related to the care continuum. • HHS OCR's enforcement also led to a California surgeon agreeing to treat patients with HIV after losing HHS funding for violating Section 504 of the Rehabilitation Act of 1973, and a Voluntary Resolution Agreement with a North Carolina assisted living facility, that agreed to change policies and procedures to accept clients living with HIV and reduce barriers to care. • DOJ began providing technical assistance during HHS OCR's on-site visit if the HHS-OCR review identified potential areas of non-compliance with Section 504 and Title III of the Americans with Disabilities Act. In addition, the DOJ-Federal Coordination and Compliance Section also indicated that they would provide technical assistance, if necessary, regarding any LEP issues that HHS-OCR identified during the on-site compliance review.

Recommendation 3: Strengthen data collection, coordination and use of data to improve health outcomes and monitor use of Federal resources

Action	Federal Agency Activities
3.1 Federal agencies will expand upon HHS efforts outlined above and harmonize HIV data collection and increase interoperability of HIV data systems to improve care continuum outcomes.	• Throughout 2014, Office of HIV/AIDS and Infectious Disease Policy (OHAIDP) worked with HRSA, CDC, SAMHSA, ONC, and OMB to improve data collection, harmonization, and sharing, reduce grantee reporting burden, and achieve greater standardization with a discrete subset of HIV data elements. ONC's Standards and Interoperability Framework is being adapted to inform and develop a monitoring system for advances in data collection across HHS. • SAMHSA and CDC are working together to align data collected for HIV testing and to reduce data collection burden by including a common set of core variables that are defined in the same way across agencies, containing fewer agency-specific variables, and eliminating data elements that are no longer essential. • IHS standardized data tracking of newly reported HIV cases at the national level as part of its effort to reduce the HIV reporting burden at the local level while improving the understanding of outcomes along the HIV Care Continuum across the agency. The 2014 national review of HIV tests showed a positivity rate of 0.1% of all HIV tests recorded by IHS. • HRSA added HIV positivity rate and Linkage to Care as core indicator to evaluate Health Center's performance. • HUD identified successful models to increase interoperability of HIV data systems from the 2011 Integrated HIV/AIDS Housing Plan SPNS grants, integrating HOPWA and Ryan White data systems in order to better assess housing's impact on the health outcomes of HOPWA program beneficiaries by developing data bridges between Homeless Management Information System and Ryan White Careware. • HRSA, with input from ONC, CMS, and OHAIDP began to format three HHS core indicators related to the HIV Care Continuum for use in the electronic medical records.

3.2 Increase technical assistance efforts to states and locally-funded jurisdictions to describe and monitor care continuums in their locales	• A CDC/HIV Surveillance grantee work group on lab data initiated monthly calls since 2013. Topics include lab reporting, testing algorithms, and assessment of completeness of lab data; these topics are related to states and locally-funded jurisdictions' ability to monitor the care continuum. • CDC has continued ongoing technical assistance by HIV surveillance Project Officers to HIV surveillance grantees on how to calculate the continuum of care using CDC technical guidance for local analyses, as well as use of data for public health follow-up to improve re-engagement in care (the Data to Care Strategy).
3.3 Require that eligibility for related HIV surveillance funding be contingent on the collection and submission of data necessary to monitor the care continuum	• CDC funded two cooperative agreements—Cooperative Re-Engagement Controlled Trial (CoRECT) and Partnerships for Care (P4C) —for which eligibility was limited based on having laws or regulations that required reporting of all CD4 and viral load test results to HIV surveillance. A core activity of both projects is the use of individual-level surveillance data for public health follow-up for engagement/re-engagement in care (a public health strategy called "Data to Care").
3.4 Support a newly funded initiative to increase states' use of continuum of care data to more effectively target public health interventions and care	• HRSA began funding a three-year SPNS Health Information Technology Capacity Building initiative for Monitoring and Improving Health Outcomes along the HIV Care Continuum, supporting four grantees awarded under the Ryan White Program Parts A or B to enhance the health information technology systems in jurisdictions by more fully integrating and utilizing relevant measures of HIV treatment, surveillance, laboratory and other program data, in order to build their own HIV care continuum. • CDC funded four state health departments under the Partnerships for Care (P4C): Health Departments and Health Centers Collaborating to Improve HIV Health Outcomes project to build sustainable partnerships with HRSA-funded health centers to support expanded HIV service delivery in communities highly affected by HIV, especially among racial and ethnic minorities. State health departments and health centers will work together to increase the identification of undiagnosed HIV infection, establish new access points for HIV care and treatment, and improve HIV outcomes along the continuum of care for people living with HIV.

Recommendation 4: Prioritize and promote research to fill gaps in knowledge along the care continuum

Action	Federal Agency Activity

4.1 Support new implementation research that takes into account the complexities of the interplay of individual behavior, social, structural, and biomedical factors on care continuum outcomes.	• VA funded over 35 Medical Centers to implement quality improvement projects along the care continuum that will be evaluated for effectiveness and potential for dissemination. The VA HIV Clinical Case Registry is monitoring and identifying gaps along the care continuum, with a particular focus on actionable intervention points, and the HIV/Hepatitis Quality Enhancement Research Initiative continues to focus their research efforts on implementation research in key areas along the HIV care continuum, to move evidence into practice to improve identification and care of Veterans with HIV and Hepatitis.
	
	• CDC funded the development and pilot testing of Positive Health Check, a computer-based intervention for use by clients with HIV in clinic waiting rooms to improve outcomes along the HIV care continuum and reduce HIV transmission risk, by providing information that is individually tailored to the patient based on his or her responses.
	
	• Following systematic literature reviews of new interventions that successfully increased linkage to HIV care, retention in HIV care, and HIV medication adherence, CDC added new interventions to the Compendium of Evidence-Based Interventions and Best Practices for HIV Prevention, which now includes nine interventions that significantly increase linkage to HIV care or retention in HIV care and ten interventions that significantly improve HIV medication adherence.
	
	• CDC funded in-depth qualitative research to assess perceived barriers and facilitators to effective patient engagement and retention in care as well as referral to other services that support patient health and well-being, and to better understand the barriers to HIV care and risk reduction in a diverse sample of HIV-positive gay and bisexual men and their serodiscordant partners.
	
	• CDC began conducting qualitative research to better understand the factors affecting the effectiveness of public health and community responses to HIV prevention and care among gay and bisexual men in local jurisdictions.
	
	• NIH initiated implementation research as a way to reduce the "implementation gap" in program delivery and by developing models that increase the public health impact of HIV prevention, treatment and care services by funding:
	  ○ HPTN 065, which will provide key information for implementation of an HIV test-and-treat strategy across the US;
	  ○ HPTN 073, designed to determine the willingness of black men who have sex with men to use a daily antiretroviral pill as pre-exposure prophylaxis.
	
	• NIH published multiple funding opportunity announcements to advance scientific research addressing the HIV care continuum:
	  ○ "Accelerating Improvements in the HIV Care Continuum" directly solicits research that will develop and test innovative strategies to reduce gaps in the HIV care continuum.
	  ○ "Strengthening Adherence to Antiretroviral-Based HIV Treatment and Prevention" seeks research to improve maintenance of viral suppression through novel antiretroviral medication adherence support programs and interventions.
	  ○ "Targeted Basic Behavioral and Social Science and Intervention Development for HIV Prevention and Care" solicits basic behavioral and social science research on barriers and facilitators of HIV care engagement to inform future intervention approaches.
	  ○ "Improving Delivery of HIV Prevention and Treatment through Implementation Science and Translational Research" calls for implementation science to evaluate health care policies, programs, and practices promoting rapid linkage to care, sustained engagement in care, and antiretroviral treatment adherence and persistence.

	• The NIH-funded inter-CFAR working group originally formed to cooperate on National HIV/AIDS Strategy goals was renamed the HIV Continuum of Care Working Group, and was expanded to include the NIMH supported HIV/AIDS Centers. • The HIV Prevention Trials Network began developing a study to assess the feasibility of a randomized trial of a community-based combination intervention to close gaps in the HIV Care Continuum and reduce new infections among MSM in the US.
4.2 Support the development and study of new HIV medication formulations and delivery systems to improve treatments and rates of virologic suppression	• NIH initiated research to support the development of new formulations and long acting antiretrovirals for HIV treatment and prevention through its basic sciences research programs, the Integrated Pre-clinical Clinical Program, and through the Microbicides Trials Network and HIV Prevention Trials Network.
4.3 Support new basic science to help advance HIV cure research.	• NIH prioritized and augmented funds and activities to support research towards a cure for HIV. As announced by the President on World AIDS Day 2013, NIH is increasing research toward a cure by $100 million over fiscal years 2015 to 2017 by shifting funds within existing resources. NIH increased research to better understand the biology of viral latency, persistence, and reservoir formation. • NIH developed cure treatment research protocols for HIV-infected newborns who will be studied through the IMPAACT Network. Adult Cure protocols are also under developed.

Recommendation 5: Provide information, resources, and technical assistance to strengthen the delivery of services along the care continuum, particularly at the state and local levels

Action	Federal Agency Activity
5.1 Develop a core curriculum requirement that teaches basic contemporary HIV concepts, with a focus on information relevant to the care continuum; this training will be required of certain Federal employees working in the HIV field, including project officers, and certain staff of Federal HIV care and prevention grant recipients.	• HHS OHAIDP in coordination with CDC, HRSA, SAMHSA, ONDCP, DOL, HUD, and VA, identified and inventoried 103 informational tools, resources, and technical assistance materials that met the following criteria: 1) Address one or more steps in the HIV care continuum; 2) respond to the needs of high priority populations; 3) have a designated steward; 4) and are appropriate for use with Federal staff and has offered recommendations to ONAP for improving training among the federal HIV workforce engaged in programmatic work.
5.2 Implement new training and technical assistance activities to increase the capacity of health departments and community-based organizations to leverage opportunities created by the Affordable Care Act to improve outcomes along the care continuum.	• The Affordable Care Act and Mental Health Parity and Addiction Equity Act are working to expand access to mental health or substance use disorders benefits and should have parity with other medical or surgical benefits. • HRSA funded the cooperative agreement: *Contracting with Medicaid and Marketplace Insurance Plans - Establishing Service Models among AIDS Service Organizations to Engage Vulnerable Populations in HIV Care Continuum Services*. • SAMHSA has begun a program in collaboration with partner agencies, ODNCP, CDC and HRSA to assist with provider training on medication-assisted treatment for opioid use disorder including trainings that will lead to physician waiver eligibility to engage in office-based treatment of opioid use disorder. SAMHSA's PCSS-MAT program facilitated these trainings and SAMHSA's Division of Pharmacologic Therapies worked collaboratively with partners to determine innovative approaches to dissemination of office-based treatment of opioid use disorder.

	• HRSA signed a cooperative agreement with Fenway Community Health Center in July, 2014 to develop training content in two domains for AIDS service organizations: organizational sustainability, and best practice models along the HIV care continuum. • Several of HRSA's national cooperative agreement partners will develop training and technical assistance opportunities for health centers to learn more about improving HIV service delivery to and HIV health outcomes for black gay and bisexual men, transgender clients, migratory and seasonal agricultural workers, people experiencing homelessness, and people living in southern states.
5.3 Develop and disseminate guidance on how both the Affordable Care Act and Medicaid expansion can be used to facilitate access to care, prevention, and supportive services for people living with HIV	• IHS educated staff on the impact of the Affordable Care Act (ACA) on IHS programs, identified the role of patient assistance programs in providing HIV and Hepatitis C medications, and described the process of helping patients obtain medication coverage through the AIDS Drugs Assistance Program. • HUD offices activated partnerships on an ACA Technical Assistance initiative for HOPWA and Homeless Continuum of Care program grantees to develop an online resource library to catalog relevant ACA resources; a searchable ACA repository of state-specific information; and ACA listserv to promote timely information to interested grantees and recipients; and the development of ACA-related fact sheets for housing providers. • In 2014, CMS and HRSA convened key advocacy and consumer agencies, including HIV/AIDS organizations to provide information regarding fiscal year 2015 enrollment activities.
5.4 Provide technical assistance and trainings to better coordinate and align the provision of housing services with medical care for people living with HIV	• HUD released a white paper explaining housing's connection to the HIV Care Continuum, and is also developing a 2015 Technical Assistance Initiative focusing on building HOPWA grantee capacity to demonstrate the link between housing and health outcomes at the local level. HUD has identified models of improved community planning, resource utilization, and service integration to better coordinate and streamline access to existing local services and resources (including medical care and other health services) for low-income persons living with HIV. • HUD is proposing a joint correspondence to all HOPWA and Ryan White grantees to convey the collaborative partnership between Federal agencies administering housing and medical resources for individuals living with HIV. More importantly, HUD has issued a white paper *entitled HIV care continuum the connections between Housing and Improved Outcomes along the HIV care continuum* as a platform for educating the intersections of housing and health and impacts of stable housing and better health outcomes which results in reduced viral transmission.
5.5 Place new emphasis on improving outcomes along the care continuum for AIDS Education and Training Centers (AETC)	• AETC grant applicants will be required to frame training activities in the context of the HIV care continuum with the intent of better educating our workforce to understand the complexities of the HIV Care Continuum and improve outcomes along each step. This emphasis will be built into the competitive funding opportunities starting this fiscal year.

V. On-the-Ground Implementation in Several Major Cities

Ongoing community engagement is a key tenet of continued National HIV/AIDS Strategy and HIV Care Continuum Initiative implementation. To directly hear from community members, frontline workers, and people living with HIV, as in years past, the Office of National AIDS Policy traveled to cities across the country and hosted a series of public listening sessions with colleagues from HHS and state and local health departments. In 2014, we visited the following locations: Jackson, Mississippi; Charleston and Columbia, South Carolina; Atlanta, Georgia; Oakland, California; San Francisco, California; Chicago, Illinois; Harlem and Brooklyn, New York.

The listening sessions reflected on the challenges and opportunities facing each region in addressing HIV in communities: to reduce new infections. The common thread uniting all of the regions was the unwavering commitment to achieve an AIDS-free generation in the United States. Even in cities where the challenges are great, there is hope that issues can be addressed and that people living with HIV will survive and thrive. Presented in the following section are programs, organizations, efforts, barriers, and assertions made by people in the cities we visited. Language in quotation marks are direct quotes from participants in the public listening sessions.

> **"I think it would be proper for us to remember to be the change that we want to see in the world, connect ourselves to one another, to live out Dr. Martin Luther King's notion of the beloved community where all stigma is removed and all individuals are returned to productivity."**
>
> — Oakland, CA listening session / June 24, 2014

Common Barriers to Care across Jurisdictions

In each locality, people living with HIV confront various barriers to accessing prevention, treatment and care services. Themes that were common across many of the regions include stigma and fear, financial barriers, and access to education and employment, and transportation. Access was identified as an issue in particular in States that have not chosen to expand Medicaid.

Addressing Barriers to Care Across the Care Continuum

While many of the barriers to care were similar across the country, the strategies that each city uses to address them vary by city. The best-practice strategies outlined below might be adapted and tailored for communities around the country.

Jackson, Mississippi:

When it comes to enacting best practices to overcome barriers to care, the word "integration" has deep meaning in Jackson. The health care community in Jackson has embraced the integration of service-delivery as a care model for treating patients with HIV. As explained by one participant, "We've got a multi-pronged approach that's going to hit statewide and certainly some of it is being supported by CAPUS (Care and Prevention in the United States) funding that really focuses on health disparities."

Like most cities, Jackson has not only established successful programs, but is sustaining them as well. **My Brother's Keeper, Inc.** is a community-based organization that is an excellent example of integration and sustainability of services and care. Another avenue that is being used in Jackson to break down barriers is a Mississippi Department of Health PSA campaign called "Be Positive You're Negative" along with the "Know It" national campaign. The campaigns feature the simple message that everyone should know their status, especially if they have risk factors.

> "I think the simple answer is you have to go to pastors and ask them. Every single one I work with, over 200 pastors here and in other parts of the country—and it's just sitting down and saying, 'Pastor I need your help. This is a public health crisis. How can we do this in a way that makes sense for you and your congregation?' It's not rocket science. It's just community mobilization, one church at a time."
>
> — Jackson, MS listening session / May 29, 2014

Given Jackson's cultural foundations, participants emphasized that the need to reach out to faith communities is critical. Organizations such as **Faith in Action** and **Open Arms Healthcare Center** have been working with churches, to spread the message that HIV/AIDS is a public health crisis and help is needed to reach members of their congregations. **Faith in Action** has convened approximately 50 faith leaders to talk about HIV and AIDS, particularly the importance of getting tested and linked to care.

The Mississippi State government and Jackson municipal government have also taken a role to break down barriers to care, including providing treatment through the ADAP, and piloting a program in Northern Mississippi to directly mail clients their medications. State officials also pointed out that it has been helpful that the Federal government has allowed states to use Ryan White money to pay co-pays, deductibles and premiums.

Columbia, South Carolina:
South Carolina has been very aggressive in engaging in social marketing campaigns to help raise awareness about HIV, particularly CDC's *Act Against AIDS* Campaign, partnership with 19 of the nation's leading African American and Latino organizations, and the "Start Talking. Stop HIV" campaign.

Atlanta, Georgia:
Underscoring the need for better coordination and less fragmentation, one participant called for a Georgia state-specific HIV/AIDS strategy to strengthen coordination and maximize the use of resources while also noting the lack of a standardized methodology for putting together a care continuum.

Another participant emphasized the need to learn more about the culture of others. **Someone Cares, Inc**. of Atlanta has implemented cultural competency trainings. A representative reported that these trainings to enhance cross-cultural relations are required to enhance care and treatment.

Oakland, California:
There are excellent examples of best practices emanating from Oakland such as the launch of a Trust Clinic to make sure that people have their basic needs taken care of before even engaging in their clinical care. The clinic has been successful in getting over 90 percent of people into stable housing. They then move into clinic care and psychiatric or mental health care as well.

> "In addition to the [New York] Department of Health's vast prevention portfolio, we implement a range of Ryan White and CDC-funded programs for persons living with HIV that intend to improve outcomes along the continuum. For example, we have extensive HIV testing programs and programs to support HIV testing, programs to support ADAP, our coordination, housing and other supportive services."
>
> — Brooklyn, NY listening session / August 8, 2014

San Francisco, CA:
For more than 30 years, San Francisco has been dealing with the fight against HIV/AIDS. In dealing with this fight, it has established several best practices including a San Francisco General Hospital model of care that engages people "in the moment", rapidly moving them from testing to care and treatment. There is also the San Francisco Department of Public Health's special emphasis on helping patients get linked to care or re-engaged in care through two unique programs that have contributed to improvements in key linkages to care indicators citywide (and exceeded the National HIV/AIDS Strategy 2015 goal).

Chicago, Illinois:
Like the other cities, Chicago has placed a great deal of time and effort into addressing the barriers facing people living with HIV. CAHISC, the Chicago Area HIV Integrated Services Council, is the new HIV planning council for the Chicago Department of Public Health, and provides guidance and feedback to the Department on the allocation of approximately $39 million in HIV prevention, care and housing dollars.

Other best practices include Chicago House, which provides not only housing services, but also started one of the nation's largest employment programs, and recently launched the TransLife Center to provide comprehensive services for the transgender community. The Chicago Black Gay Men's Caucus, established in 2005 by a group of community advocates and local health department officials, motivated by reports suggesting that black, gay and bisexual men continue to be disproportionately affected by HIV/AIDS in Chicago and the surrounding suburbs, specializes in the implementation of evidence-based HIV and STI prevention interventions, tailored specifically to the needs of this diverse group of men.

New York, New York:
ONAP held two listening sessions in New York City, one each in Harlem and Brooklyn. It was noted that Governor Andrew Cuomo had announced his commitment to end HIV/AIDS as an epidemic in New York and that he was in the process of convening a Task Force that will develop and roll-out a plan. New York has also eliminated the need for written informed consent prior to HIV testing, which has been shown to be a barrier to routine testing.

> "We cannot afford to be silent; too many have died already. We must do better with your help, with the tools provided to us by the Affordable Care Act and the National HIV/AIDS Strategy, we will."
>
> — Columbia, SC listening session / June 3, 2014

Acknowledgements

The Office of National AIDS Policy (ONAP) is grateful for the leadership and participation of the many community-based organizations, business representatives, state and local health department officials, and advocates who contributed in immeasurable ways to bring these discussions to meaningful fruition. ONAP similarly expresses gratitude to the State and local elected officials who participated in the community discussions, including Members of Congress, State representatives, and mayors. Furthermore, ONAP offers special thanks to the many people living with HIV for their courageous and frank testimony that made these discussions compelling and useful.

VI. Moving Forward

This first anniversary of the HIV Care Continuum Initiative is an opportunity to meaningfully contemplate our collective work. Much has been discussed about scientific innovation, expanded insurance coverage, and a committed Administration and Federal workforce converging to realize our ability to slow the HIV/AIDS epidemic here at home. Upon this anniversary, we are offered an opportunity to reflect on our substantial accomplishments, the places where we are called to redouble our efforts, and the ways we need to alter our approaches.

Our challenge remains complex and multi-faceted in that even as we are obliged to persist in ensuring HIV/AIDS awareness, education, and prevention occur among all Americans, we are compelled to place a laser-like focus on applying prevention, care and treatment interventions with those people and places that remain at highest risk and who face the greatest disparities in incidence, health outcomes and mortality.

For instance, researchers at Emory University and amfAR recently published a modeling study that examined to what degree differences in HIV care among black and white MSM with HIV might explain disparities in new HIV infections between HIV-negative black versus white MSM. They found that reducing racial disparities in new HIV infections among MSM cannot realistically occur by improving HIV care outcomes alone. Research into game changing prevention and care tools is needed to fundamentally reduce the racial imbalance in new HIV infections among black MSM. Ideally, these tools would include effective HIV vaccines, microbicides, as well as PrEP for HIV-negative black MSM, and a cure for all those living with HIV.[18]

The CDC reports a disturbing rise in syphilis among men of all ages while rates of gonorrhea and chlamydia remain high among young people in their teens and early 20's. Knowing that sexual transmitted infections can be a harbinger of HIV compels us to identify and eliminate these risk factors that jeopardize the health and well-being of all members of our society, and to promote the protective factors that can prevent our youth from contracting even more challenging STIs such as HIV.

Federal agencies are implementing stellar work to address the intersection of HIV/AIDS, violence against women and girls, and gender-related health disparities. An intervention that has been developed to address the trauma that many women and girls experience should be scaled up, and examined for possible adaptation and tailoring to address the trauma experienced by young gay men. Community efforts have followed the President's instruction to address this intersection for women and girls, and moving forward together, in partnership, we can bend the curve of both epidemics.

Since its beginning, the President has directed that our work remain rooted in science. As we move into 2015 and commence updating the National HIV/AIDS Strategy objectives, we will be guided by that directive as we engage Federal partners and community stakeholders in setting forth new measures. Moreover, as we work to accelerate the pace with which we collect, analyze and disseminate surveillance data, also requisite is a willingness to use it wisely, and as a tool to guide our funding, programming and policy decisions to improve outcomes along the care continuum and achieve the Strategy's goals, all in a commitment to realize the Strategy's Vision that that "the United States will become a place where new HIV infections are rare and when they do occur, every person, regardless of age, gender, race/ethnicity, sexual orientation, gender identity or socio-economic circumstance, will have unfettered access to high quality, life-extending care, free from stigma and discrimination."

---

18. Rosenberg ES, et al. Understanding the HIV disparities between black and white men who have sex with men in the USA using the HIV care continuum: a modelling study. The Lancet HIV, Early Online Publication, 18 November 2014 doi:10.1016/S2352-3018(14)00011-3.

VII. List of Acronyms

ACA	Affordable Care Act
ADAP	AIDS Drug Assistance Program
AETC	AIDS Education and Training Center
ART	Antiretroviral Therapy
CBO	Community-based organization
CDC	Centers for Disease Control and Prevention (HHS)
CFAR	Centers for AIDS Research
CMS	Centers for Medicare and Medicaid Services (HHS)
DEA	Drug Enforcement Administration
DOJ	U.S. Department of Justice
DOL	U.S. Department of Labor
FDA	Food and Drug Administration (HHS)
FQHC	Federally Qualified Health Center
HHS	U.S. Department of Health and Human Services
HOPWA	Housing Opportunities for Persons with AIDS
HPTN	HIV Prevention Trials Network (NIH)
HRSA	Health Resources and Services Administration (HHS)
HUD	U.S. Department of Housing and Urban Development
IDU	Injection Drug User
IHS	Indian Health Service (HHS)
IMPAACT	International Maternal, Pediatric, Adolescent AIDS Clinical Trials Network
IOM	Institute of Medicine
MMP	Medical Monitoring Project
MSM	Men who have sex with men
NIH	National Institutes of Health (HHS)
NIMH	National Institute of Mental Health (NIH)
OCR	Office for Civil Rights (HHS)
OHAIDP	Office of HIV/AIDS and Infectious Disease Policy (HHS)
OMB	Office of Management and Budget
ONAP	White House Office of National AIDS Policy
ONC	Office of the National Coordinator for Health Information Technology (HHS)
ONDCP	Office of National Drug Control Policy
P4C	Partnerships for Care (CDC/HRSA)
PEPFAR	U.S. President's Emergency Plan for AIDS Relief
PrEP	Pre-Exposure Prophylaxis
SAMHSA	Substance Abuse and Mental Health Services Administration (HHS)
SMAIF	Secretary's Minority AIDS Initiative Fund (HHS)
SPNS	Special Projects of National Significance (HRSA)
USTSPF	United States Preventive Services Task Force
VA	U.S. Department of Veterans Affairs

www.ingramcontent.com/pod-product-compliance
Lightning Source LLC
Chambersburg PA
CBHW052027280526
45793CB00005B/1149